BARBER FUNDAMENTALS

1 ON 1

A guide To First-time Barbers

DANIEL CHISHOLM

Contents

CHAPTER 1

INTRODUCTION TO BARBERING

This chapter dives into the exciting world of barbering, offering an in-depth look at its rich history from ancient roots to modern evolution.

Barbering's origins date back to ancient civilizations like Egypt, Mesopotamia, and the Indus Valley, where grooming was both a practical necessity and a social ritual. Egyptians used copper razors, often replacing shaved hair with elaborate wigs denoting status. Mesopotamians and Indus Valley inhabitants also had developed grooming tools, reflecting their sophisticated personal hygiene practices.

Hair held deep religious and spiritual significance. In Egypt, priests shaved their entire bodies for purity, while in Greece and India, hair was integral to religious ceremonies and social status. The rise of specialized barbers in medieval Europe saw them performing roles beyond haircuts, such as minor surgeries and dentistry, symbolized by the barber pole.

During the Renaissance, barber shops became social hubs, separating barbering from surgical practices. In Asia, barbering traditions evolved uniquely, with itinerant barbers in China and specialized tokoyama in Japan catering to samurai and geisha.

The History of Barbering: The art of barbering boasts a rich and fascinating history, stretching back millennia. This first part of our exploration delves into the earliest roots of this profession, examining how hair care evolved from a practical necessity to a social and cultural practice.

Early Civilizations (3000 BC - 476 AD)

This chapter explores hair grooming practices in ancient civilizations like Egypt, Mesopotamia, and the Indus Valley. We delve into the tools used, such as primitive razors made from flint or seashells, and the cultural significance of hair. We also examine the religious and spiritual meanings tied to hairstyles and shaving practices, which were often linked to social status and rituals. Lastly, we look at the rise of specialized barbers, who not only groomed hair but also performed roles like dentistry and minor surgery, highlighting the evolution of barbering from a practical necessity to a respected profession.

Egypt: In ancient Egypt, hair care was both an art and a necessity. Egyptians used razors made from copper and gold, and hair was often shaved off and replaced with elaborate wigs to denote status and cleanliness. Barbers were highly respected and held significant social standing.

Mesopotamia: Mesopotamians valued grooming and had a range of tools including tweezers, razors, and curling irons. Beards and hair were styled to reflect social and political status, and intricate grooming practices were common among the elite.

Indus Valley: The Indus Valley civilization also placed a high value on grooming. Archaeological findings reveal the use of small combs and razors, indicating a developed sense of personal hygiene and style.

Religious and Spiritual Significance

In ancient societies, hair carried profound religious and spiritual significance. This chapter explores how hairstyles and shaving practices were intertwined with social status, religious rites, and mourning rituals. Hairstyles often reflected one's rank or role within the community, while specific grooming practices were integral to religious ceremonies and expressions of grief. By examining these cultural connections, we gain insight into how hair was more than just a personal adornment—it was a vital element of identity and ritual in ancient times.

Ancient Egypt: Priests shaved their entire bodies, including their heads, to maintain ritual purity. Hair offerings were also made to the gods, signifying devotion and sacrifice.

Ancient Greece: In Greece, long hair was a sign of wealth and power. However, certain religious rites required the shaving of heads or beards. The god Apollo, often depicted with long flowing hair, became a symbol of youthful beauty and strength.

Ancient India: In Hindu culture, hair was a significant

element in religious ceremonies. The practice of tonsure (shaving the head) was a common ritual for monks, symbolizing renunciation of worldly possessions and ego.

The Rise of Specialized Barbers

As societies evolved, specialized barbers began to emerge, taking on more complex roles. This chapter explores the duties of these early barbers, who not only provided haircuts and shaves but also performed additional tasks such as dentistry and minor surgeries. These barbers were essential in their communities, offering a range of services beyond grooming. Their multifaceted roles highlight the growing complexity of barbering as a profession and its importance in early societies. By understanding these responsibilities, we appreciate how barbering has historically intersected with various aspects of health and social care.

Medieval Europe: During the Middle Ages, barbers were not only responsible for haircuts and shaves but also for medical procedures. Known as barber-surgeons, they performed bloodletting, tooth extractions, and minor surgeries. The barber pole, with its red and white stripes, symbolizes the blood and bandages associated with their trade.

The Renaissance: In the Renaissance period, barbering began to separate from surgical practices. Barber Shops became centers of social interaction where men gathered not only for grooming but also for news and conversation.

Asia: In China and Japan, barbering traditions developed uniquely. In China, barbers were itinerant, moving from village to village. In Japan, barbers (tokoyama) became specialized in cutting the elaborate hairstyles of samurai and geisha.

The history of barbering is a testament to its importance across different cultures and eras. From the ancient civilizations that revered hair care to the multifaceted roles of barber-surgeons, barbering has always been more than just cutting hair—it has been a reflection of societal values, religious beliefs, and cultural practices. As we move forward in this course, understanding these roots will enrich our appreciation and practice of the craft.

CHAPTER 2

BARBERING IN THE GRECO-ROMAN WORLD

The Greeks (800 BC - 146 BC)

In ancient Greece, the significance of hair and beard styles extended beyond mere aesthetics; it was a crucial aspect of identity and social status. Barbers, known as "kouris," played an integral role in Greek social life, often operating out of small shops or in public spaces where men would gather to discuss politics, philosophy, and daily affairs. These barbers were not only responsible for grooming but also served as confidants and unofficial advisors.

Greek barbers utilized a variety of tools, the most notable being the strigil, a curved, metal instrument used primarily by athletes to scrape off sweat and dirt before or after bathing. The strigil was a testament to the Greek emphasis on physical fitness and hygiene. In addition to the strigil,

Greek barbers employed razors, shears, and combs, crafted from materials such as bronze and iron. The mastery of these tools required significant skill, highlighting the barber's esteemed position in society.

Hair and beard styles were symbolic in Greek culture. The length and style of a man's hair could denote his age, status, and even his philosophical beliefs. For instance, followers of the philosopher Pythagoras were known for their distinctive long hair and beards. Meanwhile, young men typically supported shorter haircuts, which were easier to maintain and suited the athletic ideals of the time. The process of grooming was often accompanied by aromatic oils and perfumes, further emphasizing the luxurious nature of these practices.

Highly Skilled Professionals: Roman Barbering Practices

As the Greek influence waned and Rome rose to prominence, the traditions of barbering evolved but retained their central importance in daily life. Roman barbers, or "tonsors," were highly skilled professionals who catered to the grooming needs of both the elite and the common populace. The Roman obsession with cleanliness and appearance was reflected in the popularity of public baths, where many barbers set up their operations.

Roman barber shops, much like their Greek predecessors, served as social hubs where men would gather to exchange news, gossip, and discuss politics. The tonsors were adept at creating intricate hairstyles that varied significantly between different social classes and professions. For instance, Roman soldiers often wore short, practical haircuts, while the upper echelons of society favored more elaborate styles, sometimes adorned with curls and waves achieved through the use of heated metal rods.

In addition to haircuts, Roman barbering practices included the application of lotions and oils to maintain healthy hair and skin. These products were often infused with herbs and fragrances, underscoring the Roman penchant for luxury. The ritual of shaving, which was sometimes performed daily, held great significance. A clean-shaven face was seen as a mark of civilization and refinement, contrasting with the bearded "barbarians" beyond Rome's borders.

The Barber-Surgeon Guild

One of the most intriguing aspects of barbering in the Roman world was the dual role of barbers as both groomers and medical practitioners. This unique combination gave rise to the barber-surgeon, a professional who performed minor medical procedures alongside regular grooming tasks. These procedures included bloodletting, tooth extraction, and the treatment of minor wounds. The barber-surgeon's role was critical in an era when access to specialized medical care was limited.

The formation of the first barber-surgeon guilds marked a significant development in the professionalization of these roles. These guilds established standards for practice, ensuring that members were adequately trained in both barbering and surgical techniques. This dual expertise was passed down through apprenticeships, creating a lineage of skilled professionals. The legacy of the barber-surgeon would endure for centuries, influencing the development of medical and grooming practices well into the medieval period.

The dual roles of barbers in grooming and medical care underscore the multifaceted nature of their profession in ancient societies. Their contributions went beyond mere aesthetics, playing a crucial role in public health and social cohesion. As we delve deeper into the history of barbering, it becomes evident that these early practitioners laid the groundwork for a profession that would evolve and adapt to the changing needs of society.

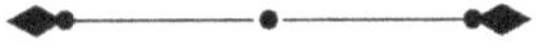

CHAPTER 3

BARBERING IN THE MIDDLE EAST AND ASIA

Islamic Traditions (610 AD - Present)

In Islamic culture, grooming and personal hygiene hold significant religious importance, guided by principles laid down in the Quran and Hadith. The Prophet Muhammad emphasized cleanliness as part of faith, leading to the development of specific haircutting and shaving practices among Muslims. For men, maintaining a beard is seen as a symbol of religious devotion, while trimming the mustache is recommended to distinguish Muslims from non-Muslims and to maintain cleanliness.

Barbers, or "halal" practitioners, in Islamic societies are often well-versed in these religious prescriptions. They perform haircuts and shaves with precision, adhering to the guidelines that dictate the permissible styles and lengths. The tools used by Islamic barbers are similar to those found in other cultures, including scissors, razors, and combs, but with an added emphasis on hygiene and ritual purity. The use of natural oils and perfumes, such as rosewater and sandalwood, is also prevalent, reflecting the Islamic tradition of using pleasant scents to maintain cleanliness and enhance personal appearance.

Islamic traditions also influence the grooming practices of women, although these are more private and varied. Women's hair is often covered in public as part of the practice of wearing hijab, but elaborate hairstyles and care routines are common within the privacy of the home. Henna, a natural dye, is frequently used to color and condition hair, adding another layer of cultural and religious significance to grooming practices.

The Art of Asian Hairdressing

Asia's diverse cultures boast a rich array of barbering traditions shaped over millennia. From China's and Japan's elaborate hairstyles to the intricate braiding techniques found in various regions, each practice reflects the unique cultural values and societal norms of its people. These traditions highlight how barbering has evolved in response to local customs, beliefs, and aesthetics, showcasing a rich heritage that continues to influence contemporary grooming practices across the continent.

China

In ancient China, hair was considered an extension of the soul and a reflection of one's moral character. Hairdressing was a revered art form, with specific styles denoting social status, marital status, and even political affiliations. For instance, during the Han Dynasty, women of the court often wore their hair in complex buns adorned with ornaments, while men sported topknots or long, flowing hair as a symbol of their scholarly pursuits.

Chinese barbers used an array of specialized tools, including combs, scissors, and hairpins made from materials like jade, gold, and ivory. The practice of hairdressing was not just about aesthetics; it was deeply intertwined with health and wellness. Traditional Chinese medicine often included scalp massages and the application of herbal treatments to promote hair growth and maintain its luster.

Japan

In Japan, the art of hairdressing reached its zenith during the Edo period, with elaborate hairstyles becoming an essential aspect of personal and social identity. The "chonmage," a topknot hairstyle, was popular among samurai and signified their warrior status. Women, especially those in the entertainment districts like geishas, wore intricate hairstyles such as the "nihongami," which required hours of careful styling and the use of waxes and combs to achieve the desired shape.

Japanese barbers and hairdressers, known as "kamiyui," were highly skilled artisans who trained for years to master their craft. The tools of their trade included delicate combs, sharp razors, and various styling aids made from natural ingredients. Hairdressing in Japan was not merely a practical task but a cultural performance, reflecting the wearer's status, profession, and personal artistry.

India

In India, hair care has been an essential part of daily life, deeply rooted in the cultural and spiritual traditions of the region. Ayurvedic practices emphasize the importance of hair care for overall health, advocating the use of natural oils like coconut and sesame oil to nourish the scalp and hair. Indian barbers, or "nai," often combined their grooming services with therapeutic treatments, offering scalp massages and herbal applications to their clients.

Hair holds significant cultural symbolism in India. For example, during certain religious ceremonies and life events, hair may be ritually cut or shaved. Sadhus, or holy men, often grow their hair long and matted as a symbol of their renunciation of worldly life, while young boys may have their heads shaved in a rite of passage known as "mundan."

Korea

In Korea, hairdressing has been influenced by various dynasties, each leaving its mark on the styles and techniques of the time. The traditional "gache" wig, worn by women during the Joseon Dynasty, was a symbol of wealth and social status. These elaborate wigs were often decorated with jewels and flowers, showcasing the wearer's affluence and attention to beauty.

Korean barbers and hairdressers utilized a range of tools and techniques to achieve the desired styles. The emphasis on natural beauty and harmony with nature was reflected in the use of organic products and meticulous grooming practices. The tradition of hairdressing in Korea has continued to evolve, blending ancient techniques with modern innovations to create unique and culturally significant styles.

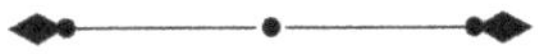

CHAPTER 4

THE ROLE OF A BARBER

The Role of a Barber: Beyond the Haircut

Barbering has evolved significantly, adapting to societal changes and trends. Today, barbers are multifaceted professionals who excel in grooming, personal care, and community building. Modern barbers master hairstyling, shaving, and beard sculpting, offering personalized hair and scalp care. Beyond technical skills, they excel in client communication, customer service, and creating welcoming environments. Barber Shops serve as community hubs, fostering social interaction. Many barbers specialize in areas like intricate designs or traditional grooming and often become entrepreneurs, opening unique shops. Embracing technology and staying updated with trends, they promote overall well being through services like scalp massages. This chapter explores these diverse roles and contributions.

Expanding Skill Sets

Hairstyling Expertise

A modern barber is a master of hairstyling, skilled in various cutting techniques such as fades, tapers, and texturizing. They are adept at creating a wide range of trendy and classic styles, tailored to the individual preferences and facial structures of their clients. This expertise requires a keen eye for detail and a deep understanding of hair types and textures. Whether it's a sleek business cut, a trendy undercut, or a timeless pompadour, a skilled barber can execute a variety of styles with precision and flair.

Shaving Specialist

The ability to deliver a clean, close shave using straight razors or safety razors is a hallmark of a skilled barber. This traditional aspect of barbering is experiencing a renaissance, with many clients seeking the classic barbershop shave experience.

Mastering the art of shaving involves understanding skin types, hair growth patterns, and the use of high-quality products to prevent irritation and achieve a smooth finish. The ritual of a hot towel shave, combined with the precise handling of a straight razor, offers a luxurious and relaxing experience that modern barbers continue to perfect.

Beard Sculpting

With the growing popularity of facial hair styles, modern barbers have become experts in beard shaping and trimming. They possess the skills to sculpt beards into various styles, from full beards and goatees to mustaches and stubble. This involves more than just trimming; it requires an understanding of facial symmetry, hair growth, and maintenance techniques. Barbers also advise clients on beard care products, such as oils and balms, to keep facial hair healthy and well-groomed.

Hair and Scalp Care

Understanding different hair types and scalp conditions allows barbers to recommend appropriate hair care products and treatments. Modern barbers are knowledgeable about the latest advancements in hair care, including shampoos, conditioners, and treatments designed to address specific issues like dandruff, dryness, or thinning hair. They provide personalized advice and solutions to help clients maintain healthy hair and scalp.

Beyond the Technical

Client Communication

Effective communication is essential for barbers, involving building rapport, listening to client needs, and offering professional advice. A good barber establishes trust and creates a comfortable environment where clients feel heard and valued. This includes asking the right questions, providing feedback, and meeting client preferences and expectations. Additionally, barbers educate clients on hair care routines and maintenance between visits, ensuring ongoing satisfaction and optimal hair health.

Customer Service Excellence

Creating a welcoming and comfortable environment, ensuring client satisfaction, and providing a positive experience are crucial to building a loyal clientele. Barber Shops often serve as safe havens where clients can relax, unwind, and enjoy a break from their daily routines. Exceptional customer service includes offering refreshments, maintaining a clean and organized space, and ensuring that each client feels appreciated and valued.

Community Hub

Barber Shops often serve as community hubs, fostering social interaction and providing a space for conversations and camaraderie. They are places where people gather to discuss local news, share stories, and build connections. Barbers play an integral role in this social dynamic, acting as confidants and friends to their clients. The barbershop environment fosters a sense of belonging and community spirit, making it a cherished institution in many neighborhoods.

Mentorship and Role Models

Experienced barbers can mentor aspiring barbers, sharing their knowledge and skills. This mentorship helps preserve the craft of barbering and ensures that high standards are maintained within the profession. By teaching the next generation of barbers, seasoned professionals contribute to the growth and sustainability of the industry. Mentorship also involves instilling values of professionalism, customer service, and continuous learning.

Specialization and Entrepreneurship

Specialization

Some barbers develop specialties within the field, focusing on areas such as men's haircuts, children's cuts, hot shaves, or intricate designs. Specialization allows barbers to refine their skills in specific areas, offering clients a level of expertise that distinguishes them from general practitioners. For instance, some barbers excel in creating detailed hair designs and patterns, while others specialize in traditional grooming techniques. This focused expertise not only enhances the quality of their services but also attracts clients seeking specific styles or treatments, thereby setting them apart in a competitive market.

Entrepreneurship

Many barbers choose to open their barbershops, allowing them to create a unique atmosphere and cater to a specific clientele. Entrepreneurship in barbering involves more than just cutting hair; it includes managing a business, marketing services, and creating a brand identity. Independent barber shops often reflect the personality and vision of their owners, offering clients a distinctive experience that combines professional grooming with a personalized touch.

The Evolving Role

Adapting to Trends

Modern barbers continuously stay updated with the latest industry trends and techniques, constantly learning and refining their skills. This adaptability allows them to meet evolving client preferences and remain competitive in the market. Continuous education through workshops, courses, and industry events is crucial for barbers to stay ahead of the curve. By embracing new styles and advancements, barbers can provide cutting-edge services and maintain a high standard of excellence. This commitment to ongoing learning ensures that they not only meet but exceed client expectations, securing their place as top professionals in the field.

Embracing Technology

Online booking systems and social media marketing are essential tools for modern barbers to connect with clients and grow their business. Technology simplifies the appointment scheduling process, making it more convenient for clients to book services.

Additionally, it allows barbers to showcase their work online, attracting new customers. Social media platforms serve as powerful marketing tools, enabling barbers to promote their services, share client testimonials, and build a dedicated following. By leveraging these digital tools, barbers can enhance their client experience, improve service visibility, and establish a strong online presence, ultimately contributing to business growth and client loyalty.

Promoting Wellbeing

Some barbers incorporate elements of scalp massage and stress reduction techniques into their services, promoting overall client wellbeing. These additional services create a holistic grooming experience that addresses both physical appearance and mental relaxation. The inclusion of scalp massages, aromatherapy, and calming environments transforms a simple haircut or shave into a rejuvenating experience.

This exploration of the modern barber's role highlights their multifaceted contribution to society. From hairstyling expertise to fostering community spirit, barbers play a vital role in the lives of their clients. Their ability to adapt, innovate, and provide exceptional service ensures that the profession remains dynamic and relevant in the modern world.

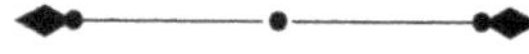

CHAPTER 5

THE BARBERING INDUSTRY TODAY

The Barbering Industry Today: A Booming Business with a Bright Future

The barbering industry is witnessing a remarkable resurgence, fueled by increasing demand for skilled barbers and a renewed focus on men's grooming. This chapter examines the contemporary landscape of barbering, highlighting key trends, addressing challenges, and uncovering exciting opportunities for professionals in the field. From the rise of intricate styles and personalized grooming experiences to the impact of technological advancements and the importance of continuing education, this chapter provides a comprehensive overview of the dynamic factors shaping the industry today.

Market Growth and Trends

Increased Demand

The demand for skilled barbers is experiencing a significant upswing, driven by a heightened awareness of men's grooming and a growing desire for personalized hair care experiences. As men become increasingly conscious of their appearance and the importance of professional grooming, the need for expert barbering services has surged. This trend is not confined to urban areas; even smaller towns and rural communities are witnessing a rise in the popularity of barbershops.

Modern men are seeking more than just a haircut; they want tailored grooming experiences that reflect their personal style and preferences. This shift has led to a boom in the barbering industry, with a growing number of barbershops offering specialized services such as beard sculpting, intricate fades, and classic cuts with contemporary twists. The revival of traditional barbering techniques, combined with innovative styling approaches, has further fueled this demand.

Moreover, the rise of social media and the influence of style icons have played a crucial role in popularizing grooming trends and making barbershops a go-to destination for the modern man. As a result, the barbering industry is thriving, offering promising opportunities for skilled barbers to cater to an ever-expanding clientele seeking high-quality, personalized grooming services.

Emerging Trends

Popular trends such as beard sculpting, intricate fades, and classic cuts with modern twists are driving client interest. These styles require a high level of skill and creativity, pushing barbers to continually improve their techniques. Additionally, the influence of social media and celebrity styles has a significant impact, as clients often seek to emulate the looks of their favorite public figures.

Diversification of Clientele

The barbering industry is no longer restricted to just men. Women seeking shorter styles and those desiring a more personalized experience are increasingly opting for barbershops. This diversification has expanded the market, creating new opportunities for barbers to showcase their versatility and attract a broader clientele.

Technological Integration

The integration of technology is transforming how barbers reach and connect with clients. Online booking systems simplify appointment scheduling, while social media marketing helps barbers showcase their work and attract new customers. Additionally, the rise of barbering apps offers tools for client management, loyalty programs, and even virtual consultations, enhancing the overall customer experience.

Challenges and Opportunities

With the rising number of barbershops and barbering schools, competition for clients is intensifying. However, barbers who carve out a niche or build strong customer loyalty can still thrive in this competitive landscape. Specializing in specific areas, such as vintage cuts, beard sculpting, or eco-friendly grooming products, can distinguish a barber from the rest.

Developing a unique style or focus allows barbers to cater to specific client preferences and needs, creating a loyal customer base. For instance, offering services with a commitment to sustainability can attract environmentally conscious clients. Similarly, mastering vintage hairstyles or intricate fades can draw in clients seeking those particular looks.

Moreover, exceptional customer service and personalized experiences are key to retaining clients. Building rapport, understanding individual preferences, and consistently delivering high-quality results foster strong relationships and encourage repeat business.

Marketing strategies, such as showcasing unique skills on social media platforms, can also enhance visibility and attract a broader audience. By leveraging these approaches, barbers can effectively differentiate themselves, overcome competition, and secure a thriving business. In an industry where trends and client expectations constantly evolve, adaptability and a distinct identity are crucial for sustained success.

Licensing and Regulations

Each state has specific licensing requirements for barbers. Understanding and adhering to these regulations is crucial for success. Navigating the complexities of state and local laws can be daunting, but compliance ensures legitimacy and professionalism. Additionally, staying informed about changes in regulations helps barbers avoid legal issues and maintain their business operations smoothly.

Continuing Education

Staying updated with the latest trends and techniques through workshops, online courses, and professional development programs is essential for maintaining a competitive edge. Continuous learning not only enhances a barber's skill set but also demonstrates a commitment to excellence. Investing in education can lead to higher client satisfaction and repeat business.

Career Paths and Earning Potential

Salary Ranges

Salaries for barbers vary widely based on experience, location, and work environment. Barbers can earn a base salary, commissions on services, or a combination of both. In bustling metropolitan areas, experienced barbers often command higher fees due to the larger clientele and higher cost of services. These barbers can capitalize on the increased demand and diverse customer preferences, which allow for premium pricing and the opportunity to build a reputation as top-tier professionals.

Conversely, barbers in smaller towns may rely more on cultivating a loyal customer base. While the fees might be lower compared to urban counterparts, the emphasis on personalized service and community relationships can foster steady business. These barbers often become integral parts of their local communities, providing a personal touch that encourages repeat clients and referrals.

Work environments also influence earnings. Barbers employed in high-end salons or upscale barber shops may enjoy additional benefits and a steady flow of clients, while independent barbers or those renting chairs might benefit from flexible schedules and greater control over their pricing and services.

Overall, the barbering profession offers diverse opportunities for earning potential, influenced by strategic location choices, skill development, and the ability to build and maintain strong client relationships.

Benefits and Ownership

Some barber shops offer benefits packages, including health insurance and retirement plans, while others may provide opportunities for commission-based earnings or even ownership for experienced barbers. Ownership or partnership in a barbershop allows barbers to share in the profits and make business decisions, offering greater financial rewards and career satisfaction.

Flexible Work Options

Independent barbers or those working in commission-based settings can often tailor their work schedules to fit their needs. This flexibility appeals to those seeking a better work-life balance or pursuing additional ventures. Freelance barbers can also work at multiple locations or offer mobile services, expanding their client base and income potential.

The Future of Barbering

Technology's Impact

The ongoing integration of technology is poised to significantly shape the barbering industry. Advancements in online booking, client management systems, and marketing tools are streamlining operations and enhancing the client experience. For instance, online booking systems simplify scheduling, reduce wait times, and improve overall convenience for both barbers and clients.

Emerging technologies like augmented reality (AR) and virtual reality (VR) are revolutionizing how clients choose hairstyles. AR and VR can allow clients to visualize different styles and cuts on themselves before making a decision, leading to greater satisfaction and reducing the risk of dissatisfaction with the final result.

Moreover, artificial intelligence (AI)-driven analytics offer barbers valuable insights into client preferences and behaviors. By analyzing data on past appointments, product purchases, and style choices, barbers can tailor their services to better meet individual client needs. This personalization not only enhances client satisfaction but also fosters loyalty and repeat business.

In addition, technology-driven marketing tools enable barbers to reach a broader audience through targeted advertising and social media engagement. By leveraging these tools, barbers can effectively promote their unique skills and services, attracting new clients and maintaining a competitive edge in a dynamic industry. Overall, embracing technological advancements will be key to future success in barbering.

Sustainability and Eco-Friendly Practices

The growing awareness of environmental consciousness is influencing the barbering industry. Sustainable practices like using eco-friendly products, reducing waste, and incorporating green building designs in barbershops will likely become increasingly important. Barbers who adopt these practices can attract environmentally conscious clients and contribute to a healthier planet.

Specialization and Niche Markets

Specialization within the barbering industry is expected to continue, with barbers focusing on specific clientele (children, athletes, etc.) or services (straight razor shaves, beard sculpting). This targeted approach allows barbers to develop expertise in particular areas, offering unique services that meet the specific needs of their clients. Niche markets can lead to increased client loyalty and higher earnings.

The Journey Ahead

The barbering industry is a dynamic and exciting field with a promising future. By staying updated with trends, honing their skills, and adapting to changing consumer preferences, barbers can ensure their success and contribute to the continued growth of this vibrant profession. The journey to becoming a barber involves several key steps:

1. **Education**: Enroll in a reputable barbering school to learn the fundamentals of hair cutting, styling, and grooming.

2. **Licensing**: Meet the licensing requirements for your state, which may include passing written and practical exams.

3. **Building Your Network**: Develop relationships with other professionals in the industry, attend trade shows, and engage in online communities to stay connected and informed.

4. **Gaining Experience**: Work in different settings, such as traditional barbershops, salons, or as a freelance barber, to gain diverse experience and refine your skills.

5. **Continuing Education**: Participate in ongoing training and professional development to stay current with industry trends and techniques.

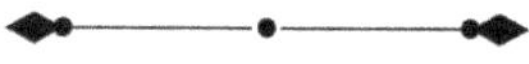

CHAPTER 6

UNDERSTANDING TOOLS AND EQUIPMENT

Mastery of tools and equipment is crucial in barbering. This chapter delves into the essential tools every barber needs, detailing their types, uses, maintenance, and selection criteria. By understanding and effectively managing clippers, guards, scissors, shears, combs, brushes, and additional tools, barbers can provide high-quality services and ensure client satisfaction. Proper tool care and selection not only enhance cutting precision and efficiency but also build a strong foundation for a successful and reputable barbering career.

Clippers and Guards

Types of Clippers

- **Magnetic vs. Detachable:** Magnetic clippers use an electromagnetic motor, ideal for lighter, quick trims, while detachable clippers feature interchangeable blades for more versatile and heavy-duty cutting.

- **Corded vs. Cordless:** Corded clippers offer consistent power but limit mobility, whereas cordless clippers provide flexibility but require regular charging.

Understanding Clipper Guards

- **Guard Sizes and Lengths:** Different guard sizes correspond to specific hair lengths, allowing for a range of styles from close cuts to longer trims.

- **Material and Quality:** Guards made from high-quality plastic or metal ensure durability and a smoother cutting experience.

- **Fading and Blending Guards:** These specialized guards create smooth transitions between hair lengths, essential for professional-looking fades and blends.

Selecting the Right Clippers and Guards

- **Matching Clippers and Guards:** Ensure that your clippers are compatible with the guards you choose.

- **Power and Performance:** Select clippers with sufficient power for your clientele's hair types, especially if dealing with thick or coarse hair.

- **Budget and Needs:** Balance your budget with your specific barbering needs, investing in high-quality tools where necessary.

Maintaining Your Clippers and Guards

- **Cleaning and Lubrication:** Regular cleaning and lubrication prevent wear and ensure smooth operation.

- **Replacing Blades and Guards:** Replace dull blades and worn-out guards to maintain cutting precision.

- **Storage and Organization:** Keep your tools organized to prevent damage and ensure efficiency.

Scissors and Shears

Types of Barber Scissors and Shears

- **Straight Shears:** Ideal for blunt cuts, precise lines, and clean finishes.

- **Offset Shears:** Popular for slicing and texturizing techniques due to their ergonomic design.

- **Thinning Shears:** Used to remove bulk and create texture without significantly reducing hair length.
- **Texturizing Shears:** Feature deeper grooves for more dramatic texturizing effects.

Choosing the Right Scissors and Shears

- **Material and Quality:** High-quality scissors are often made from Japanese stainless steel, known for its durability and sharpness.
- **Finger Hole Styles:** Choose scissors that fit comfortably, with options for different finger sizes and preferences.

Scissors and Shears Handling Techniques

- **Proper Posture:** Maintain good posture to prevent fatigue and ensure precision.
- **Finger Placement:** Correct placement of thumb and fingers in the scissor holes is crucial for control.
- **Scissor Stance:** Different stances are used for various cutting techniques, enhancing accuracy and efficiency.

Maintaining Your Scissors and Shears

- **Cleaning and Sharpening:** Regular cleaning and professional sharpening maintain cutting quality.

- **Storage:** Proper storage protects scissors from damage and dulling.

- **Signs of Dullness:** Identify dull blades by the pulling or dragging sensation during cuts.

Combs and Brushes

Types of Combs and Brushes

- **Barber Combs:** Includes cutting combs, detangling combs, afro combs, and fading combs, each designed for specific purposes.

- **Styling Brushes:** Various shapes and bristle types cater to different hair textures and styling needs.

- **Fading Brushes:** Used to blend sections during fading techniques for a seamless finish.

Choosing the Right Combs and Brushes

- **Material and Quality:** Durable materials ensure long-lasting performance.

- **Tooth Spacing and Bristle Type:** Match combs and brushes to hair types and desired outcomes.

- **Size and Comfort:** Select tools that are comfortable and balanced in hand for better control.

Combs and Brushes Techniques

- **Combining Techniques:** Proper techniques for detangling, sectioning, and directing hair flow are essential.

- **Brushing Techniques:** Learn methods for smoothing hair, creating volume, and applying styling products.

- **Using Combs and Brushes with Clippers and Shears:** Master how these tools complement each other to achieve precise cuts and blending.

Maintaining Your Combs and Brushes

- **Cleaning and Disinfection:** Regular cleaning ensures hygiene and prevents product buildup.

- **Detangling Brushes:** Periodically remove accumulated hair from bristles to maintain effectiveness.

- **Replacing Combs and Brushes:** Replace when they no longer function effectively or provide a proper grip.

Additional Tools

Essential Additional Tools

- **Clipper and Shear Oil:** Reduces friction and maintains blade sharpness with regular use.

- **Disinfectant Spray and Wipes:** Maintain a clean and hygienic workspace to ensure client safety.

- **Barber Cape and Client Gown:** Protect clients' clothing from hair clippings and styling products.

- **Spray Bottle:** Essential for dampening hair during cutting and styling.

- **Neck Strip:** Provides additional comfort and hygiene during haircuts.

- **Styling Products:** Offer a selection of high-quality styling products tailored to client needs.

- **Clipper Guards Organizer:** Keep clipper guards organized for easy access.

- **Clipper Stand:** Helps maintain a clean and organized workspace.

- **Hand Mirror:** Allows clients to view the back of their haircut during consultations and styling.

Optional Tools for Specialized Services

- **Straight Razor:** For traditional wet shaves and detailed finishing.

- **Hot Lather Machine:** Provides a luxurious shaving experience with warm lather.

- **Beard Trimmer:** Essential for detailed beard shaping and trimming.

- **Scalp Massager:** Offers a relaxing service for clients.

- **Hair Dryer:** Useful for drying and styling hair post-haircut.

Selecting and Maintaining Additional Tools

- **Invest in Quality:** Choose well-made tools for durability and reliability.

- **Prioritize Hygiene:** Regularly replace disposable items and disinfect reusable tools to maintain a clean environment.

- **Proper Storage:** Store tools in a designated area to keep them organized and readily accessible.

By understanding and properly maintaining your tools and equipment, you can ensure that you provide the highest quality service to your clients. The right tools, combined with proper techniques and care, will set the foundation for a successful and reputable barbering career.

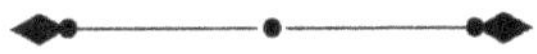

CHAPTER 7

BARBER SHOPS ANITATION: CLIENT HYGIENE AND BLOOD BORNE PATHOGENS

Building on the general barbershop sanitation principles from Part 1, this chapter focuses on client hygiene and protocols for handling bloodborne pathogens. Maintaining a safe and hygienic environment in the barbershop is crucial for protecting both clients and barbers from health risks. Topics include polite health inquiries, handling visible skin conditions, and educating clients on personal hygiene. The chapter also covers understanding bloodborne pathogens, implementing universal precautions, using personal protective equipment, and ensuring proper sharps disposal and spill response. Client cooperation and open communication are emphasized to maintain a clean and safe barbershop environment.

Client Screening and Communication

Health Inquiries: Although barbers cannot request detailed medical histories, they can engage in polite inquiries about any contagious conditions or recent illnesses that may pose a health risk during the haircutting process. Simple questions like, "Have you been feeling well recently?" or "Do you have any skin irritations we should be aware of?" can help gauge potential risks without intruding on personal privacy.

Visible Skin Conditions: If a client presents with visible skin conditions such as open wounds, rashes, or excessive flaking, barbers should professionally and courteously decline service. It's essential to explain that such conditions could compromise the cleanliness and safety of the barbershop environment. Recommending that the client seek medical attention first not only ensures safety but also demonstrates care and professionalism.

Client Education: Educating clients about the importance of personal hygiene before a haircut is crucial. Clients should be encouraged to arrive with clean hair and scalp, free of excessive dirt, product buildup, or lice. Barbers can create informative materials or posters that highlight these hygiene practices, ensuring clients understand the role they play in maintaining a sanitary environment.

Bloodborne Pathogens and Barbershop Safety

Understanding Bloodborne Pathogens: Bloodborne pathogens are infectious microorganisms in human blood that can cause diseases in humans. Examples include Hepatitis B, Hepatitis C, and HIV. Understanding these pathogens is the first step in implementing effective safety protocols in the barbershop.

Universal Precautions: The concept of universal precautions is essential in barbershop safety. This approach involves treating all blood and bodily fluids as potentially infectious, regardless of a client's known health status. By adhering to universal precautions, barbers can ensure consistent safety measures are in place for every client interaction.

Personal Protective Equipment (PPE): The use of PPE is vital in preventing the transmission of bloodborne pathogens. Barbers should wear disposable gloves during haircuts, especially when performing services like shaving or using straight razors. Additionally, eye protection may be necessary for certain procedures to protect against splashes or sprays of bodily fluids.

Sharps Safety: Handling sharp instruments like razors and blades with extreme caution is crucial. Barbers must dispose of these items in designated sharps containers immediately after use to prevent accidental cuts and injuries. These containers should be puncture-resistant and clearly labeled to ensure safe disposal.

Spill Response: Developing a comprehensive spill response plan is essential. Barber Shops should have disinfectant solutions, absorbent materials, and proper waste disposal procedures readily available to address blood spills or other bodily fluid contamination promptly. Training staff on these procedures ensures quick and effective responses to any incidents.

Barbershop Safety Protocols

Sharps Disposal: Investing in a designated sharps container specifically designed for the safe disposal of razors, blades, and other sharp objects is non-negotiable. Proper sharps disposal prevents injuries and ensures compliance with health and safety regulations.

Disinfection Procedures: Establishing clear procedures for disinfecting surfaces, tools, and equipment after each client is critical. Barbers should focus on areas that may have come into contact with blood or bodily fluids. Using EPA-approved disinfectants and following manufacturer guidelines ensures thorough sanitation.

First-Aid Kit: Maintaining a well-stocked first-aid kit in the barbershop is essential for addressing minor cuts, scrapes, or allergic reactions promptly. Barbers should be familiar with the contents of the kit and know how to use them effectively.

Vaccinations: Considering vaccinations, such as the Hepatitis B vaccine, offers an additional layer of protection for barbers. Since Hepatitis B is a common bloodborne pathogen, vaccination helps safeguard barbers against potential exposure.

Importance of Client Cooperation

Client Responsibility: Educating clients about their role in maintaining a hygienic environment is crucial. Clients should disclose any relevant health conditions and arrive for appointments with clean hair and scalp. This cooperation helps ensure a safe and pleasant experience for everyone.

Open Communication: Encouraging open communication with clients about their health status and any concerns they may have fosters a trusting relationship. Clients should feel comfortable discussing their needs and any potential risks, knowing that their barber prioritizes their safety and well-being.

By implementing these comprehensive hygiene and safety protocols, barbers can create a clean and secure environment for their clients, protecting both themselves and their clientele from health risks associated with bloodborne pathogens and poor hygiene practices.

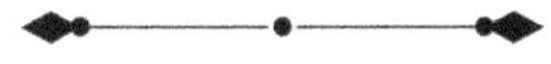

CHAPTER 8

BARBER SHOPS ANITATION: WASTE DISPOSAL AND ENVIRONMENTAL RESPONSIBILITY

Building on the foundations of general sanitation and client hygiene, this chapter explores proper waste disposal practices in a barbershop. Responsible waste disposal is essential for maintaining a clean and hygienic environment and showcases the barbershop's commitment to environmental responsibility. Topics include managing hair clippings, disposable items, and sanitation products, with a focus on recycling and composting when possible. Minimizing waste generation through reusable supplies, refillable dispensers, and energy-efficient practices is also emphasized. Proper waste disposal not only reduces environmental impact but also leads to cost savings and attracts eco-conscious clients, promoting a sustainable and positive image for the barbershop.

Types of Barbershop Waste

Hair Clippings: Hair clippings are the most common form of waste in a barbershop, resulting from haircuts and trims.

Disposable Items: This category includes used capes, gloves, masks, razors, blades, and other single-use items utilized during haircuts and styling.

Sanitation Products: Empty disinfectant spray bottles, wipes, and other sanitation products used for cleaning and disinfection contribute to barbershop waste.

Other Waste: General waste like paper towels, tissues, and coffee cups also needs proper disposal.

Proper Disposal Practices

Hair Clippings: Hair clippings can be composted if they are free of chemicals or dyes. Composting hair clippings reduces waste and enriches soil. Alternatively, bag and dispose of them in the general waste bin. Some salons partner with hair donation programs that accept clean hair clippings for charitable purposes, such as making wigs for cancer patients.

Disposable Items: Always dispose of items like gloves, masks, and razors in designated bins lined with appropriate liners. These items should not be placed in recycling bins due to contamination risks. Sharps containers should be used for razors and blades to prevent injury.

Sanitation Products: Dispose of empty disinfectant containers and wipes according to local regulations. Some may require special handling due to the chemicals they contain. Proper disposal prevents chemical contamination and ensures safety.

Other Waste: Recycle paper products like cardboard boxes and magazines whenever possible. Dispose of food waste and other organic materials in designated compost bins to reduce landfill waste.

Minimizing Waste Generation

Reusable Supplies: Use reusable barber capes and gowns instead of disposables whenever practical. Launder them regularly to maintain hygiene and reduce waste.

High-Quality Tools: Invest in durable, high-quality metal clippers and shaving mugs. These items have a longer lifespan and reduce the need for frequent replacements.

Refillable Dispensers: Opt for refillable dispensers for disinfectant solutions and cleaning products instead of individual bottles. This reduces plastic waste and is more economical in the long run.

Environmental Responsibility

Energy Efficiency: Utilize energy-efficient lighting and appliances to reduce energy consumption. LED bulbs and ENERGY STAR-rated appliances can significantly lower energy usage.

Water Conservation: Install low-flow faucets and showerheads to minimize water usage during shampooing and cleaning. Efficient water use reduces costs and conserves valuable resources.

Recycling: Develop a clear recycling system in the barbershop. Label bins for paper, plastic, and metal recycling and educate staff and clients on proper recycling practices.

Encouraging recycling helps reduce waste and supports environmental sustainability.

Benefits of Responsible Waste Disposal

Environmental Impact: Proper waste disposal practices minimize the barbershop's environmental footprint, contributing to a more sustainable future. Reducing waste and promoting recycling can significantly lessen the environmental impact of barbershop operations.

Cost Savings: Reducing reliance on disposable items and implementing reusable alternatives can lead to cost savings over time. Investing in durable, high-quality tools and refillable products reduces the frequency of purchases and waste disposal costs.

Positive Image: Demonstrating a commitment to responsible waste disposal showcases the barbershop's environmental consciousness, attracting eco-conscious clients. An environmentally responsible barbershop can differentiate itself in the market and build a loyal client base that values sustainability.

Implementing a Sustainable Barbershop

Staff Training: Educate staff on proper waste disposal practices and the importance of environmental responsibility. Regular training sessions can ensure that all employees are knowledgeable and committed to sustainability initiatives.

Client Engagement: Involve clients in your sustainability efforts. Display informative posters about your waste disposal practices and encourage clients to participate in recycling and waste reduction. Offering incentives for clients who bring reusable items, such as coffee cups, can foster a community of environmentally conscious individuals.

Continuous Improvement: Regularly assess and improve waste disposal and environmental practices. Stay updated on new sustainability trends and technologies that can further reduce the barbershop's environmental impact.

By following these guidelines for proper waste disposal and embracing practices that minimize waste generation, barber shops can operate in an environmentally responsible manner while maintaining a clean and hygienic environment. Small changes in daily habits can have a significant impact on the environment, contributing to a more sustainable future for everyone.

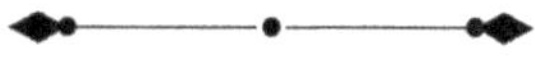

CHAPTER 9

BARBER PERSONAL HYGIENE

A barber's personal hygiene is crucial for the cleanliness, professionalism, and success of a barbershop. It fosters client trust and confidence, setting a high standard for the entire establishment. Essential hygiene practices include regular showering, wearing clean uniforms, grooming hair and beards, and maintaining good oral hygiene. Frequent handwashing, avoiding strong fragrances, and limiting jewelry are also important. Barbers should project a clean, professional image through neat attire and positive body language. By adhering to these practices, barbers contribute to a healthy, inviting environment that enhances the overall barbershop experience.

Daily Practices

Showering and Bathing: Regular showering or bathing is fundamental for maintaining cleanliness. A fresh start to the day ensures that barbers feel confident and presentable.

Clean Clothes and Uniforms: Barbers should wear clean, professional clothing, including a designated barber uniform if applicable. Uniforms should be laundered regularly to prevent the accumulation of hair, oils, and other contaminants. Investing in multiple sets of uniforms allows for daily changes, maintaining a consistently professional appearance.

Hair and Beard Maintenance: Neatly groomed hair and well-maintained beards reflect a barber's attention to detail and professionalism. Regular trims and appropriate styling prevent a disheveled appearance and promote a polished look.

Oral Hygiene: Good oral hygiene is essential for maintaining fresh breath and a professional appearance. Brushing teeth twice daily, flossing, and using mouthwash help prevent bad breath and dental issues, ensuring confidence in close interactions with clients.

Handwashing: Frequent handwashing with soap and water is crucial, especially before and after each client, and after handling dirty tools or equipment. Proper handwashing techniques involve scrubbing all parts of the hands, including between fingers and under nails, for at least 20 seconds.

Fragrances: Barbers should avoid strong perfumes or colognes that may be irritating to clients with allergies or sensitivities. Opting for mild, neutral scents or unscented personal care products helps create a comfortable environment for all clients.

Jewelry: Excessive jewelry can be unhygienic and pose a risk of snagging on hair or equipment. Limiting jewelry to minimal, simple pieces ensures safety and maintains a professional appearance.

Overall Presentation: Projecting a clean, professional image through neat attire, good posture, and positive body language enhances the client experience. A confident, well-groomed barber sets a positive tone for the barbershop.

Enhancing Professionalism Through Personal Hygiene

Nail Care: Keeping nails clean, trimmed, and free of dirt is essential. Long or dirty nails can harbor bacteria and create an unprofessional appearance. Regularly maintaining nail hygiene demonstrates attention to detail and cleanliness.

Skin Care: Healthy skin is a reflection of good hygiene practices. Using appropriate skincare products to manage oily skin, dryness, or other skin conditions helps maintain a professional appearance. Avoiding excessive use of products that may cause irritation or allergies is also important.

Footwear: Comfortable, clean, and professional footwear is crucial for barbers who spend long hours on their feet. Proper footwear not only ensures personal comfort but also contributes to the overall professional appearance.

Hygiene Breaks: Scheduling regular hygiene breaks throughout the day allows barbers to freshen up, wash hands, and ensure they maintain high hygiene standards.

These breaks also provide an opportunity to relax and reset, promoting overall well-being.

Promoting a Hygienic Work Environment

Tool and Equipment Sanitation: Regularly cleaning and disinfecting tools and equipment is vital for preventing cross-contamination and ensuring client safety. Barbers should follow established protocols for sanitizing combs, scissors, clippers, and other tools after each use.

Workstation Cleanliness: Maintaining a clean and organized workstation reflects a commitment to hygiene and professionalism. Regularly wiping down surfaces, disposing of waste promptly, and organizing tools contribute to a tidy and efficient workspace.

Personal Protective Equipment (PPE): Utilizing PPE, such as gloves and masks, when necessary, enhances hygiene and protects both barbers and clients. Proper use and disposal of PPE are critical to maintaining a safe environment.

Client Interaction: Professional hygiene extends to client interactions. Barbers should always greet clients with clean hands, maintain a pleasant demeanor, and ensure their personal hygiene does not detract from the client experience. Listening to client preferences regarding fragrances and sensitivity to products shows attentiveness and respect.

Benefits of Adhering to Personal Hygiene Practices

Client Trust and Loyalty: Consistently high personal hygiene standards foster client trust and confidence. Clients are more likely to return to a barbershop where they feel assured of the barber's cleanliness and professionalism.

Health and Safety: Maintaining personal hygiene protects barbers from potential health issues, such as infections and skin conditions, and reduces the risk of spreading illnesses to clients.

Professional Reputation: A barber's personal hygiene significantly impacts their professional reputation. A clean, well-groomed appearance enhances credibility and can attract a broader clientele, including those who prioritize hygiene and professionalism.

Workplace Morale: A hygienic work environment contributes to overall workplace morale. Barbers who take pride in their personal hygiene set a positive example for colleagues, fostering a culture of cleanliness and professionalism within the barbershop.

By adhering to these personal hygiene practices, barbers can contribute to a clean and healthy environment for themselves, their clients, and the overall barbershop experience. Personal hygiene is not only a reflection of individual professionalism but also a cornerstone of a successful, reputable barbershop.

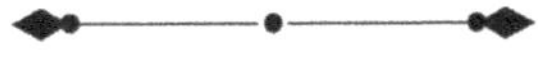

CHAPTER 10

CLIENT COMMUNICATION

Effective communication is key to building a loyal clientele. This chapter emphasizes conducting thorough consultations, actively listening to clients, understanding their expectations, and providing professional advice. Key practices include a warm welcome, active listening, and positive communication. Barbers should discuss desired haircuts, assess hair history, consider lifestyle and maintenance, and recommend suitable products. Visual aids help clarify client preferences, and professional input ensures the best outcomes. Regular follow-ups, encouraging feedback, and handling dissatisfaction professionally build trust and long-term relationships. Mastering these skills ensures client satisfaction and contributes to the barbershop's success.

Building Rapport and Understanding Client Needs

The consultation is a fundamental part of the barbering process. It involves a detailed discussion between the barber and client to clarify expectations, explore desired styles, and ensure the final haircut meets the client's needs and preferences. This process helps in understanding the client's vision, assessing their hair type and history, and providing tailored recommendations. Effective consultations build trust, allow for clear communication, and ensure client satisfaction by aligning the barber's skills with the client's goals.

Building Rapport

Warm Welcome: Greet the client with a friendly smile and introduce yourself by name.

A warm welcome sets a positive tone for the entire experience.

Active Listening: Pay close attention to the client's words, both verbal and nonverbal. Listen to their desired hairstyle, hair care routine, and any concerns they may have. Active listening involves nodding, maintaining eye contact, and occasionally repeating back what the client has said to confirm understanding.

Positive Communication: Maintain a positive and professional demeanor throughout the consultation. Use clear, concise language and avoid barber jargon that the client may not understand. Positive communication builds trust and makes clients feel valued.

Understanding Client Needs

Desired Haircut: Discuss the specific haircut the client is interested in. Ask them to show you reference pictures if available. Visual aids can significantly help in understanding their vision and ensuring satisfaction.

Hair History and Growth Patterns: Inquire about the client's hair history, including previous haircuts, styling habits, and any hair growth concerns they may have. Understanding their hair type, texture, and growth patterns will influence the haircut recommendation.

Lifestyle and Maintenance: Consider the client's lifestyle and how much time they are willing to dedicate to hair care and styling. Recommend styles that fit their daily routine and maintenance capabilities. This ensures the client can easily manage their new look.

Hair Products: Discuss the client's current hair care products and styling routine. Offer recommendations for products that will complement the chosen haircut. Tailored product advice can enhance the client's hair health and styling ease.

Conducting Thorough Consultations

Step-by-Step Consultation Process

Greeting and Introduction: Start with a warm greeting and introduce yourself. Make the client feel comfortable and valued from the beginning.

Assessment: Begin by assessing the client's current hairstyle, hair condition, and scalp health. This initial evaluation provides a foundation for the consultation.

Client Preferences: Ask open-ended questions about the client's desired style, daily hair care routine, and any specific issues they face with their hair. Encourage them to share as much detail as possible.

Visual Aids: Use mirrors, magazines, or digital devices to show different styles and get a clear idea of the client's preferences. Visual references help bridge the gap between what the client envisions and what is achievable.

Professional Input: Based on the client's input, offer your professional advice. Explain why certain styles may or may not work with their hair type or lifestyle. Offer alternative suggestions that align with their preferences.

Agreement: Ensure both you and the client are on the same page before proceeding. Confirm the final decision on the style and any additional services like shampooing, conditioning, or beard trimming.

Offering Professional Advice

Customized Recommendations

Styling Techniques: Educate clients on how to style their hair at home. Demonstrate techniques that are easy to replicate and provide tips for maintaining the salon look.

Product Knowledge: Share your knowledge about hair care products that suit their hair type and style. Explain the benefits of each product and how to use them effectively.

Hair Health Tips: Advice on maintaining hair health, such as regular trims, proper washing techniques, and the importance of using heat protection when styling.

Aftercare Instructions: Provide detailed aftercare instructions to ensure the client can maintain their new look until their next visit. This might include how often to wash their hair, which products to use, and how to style it daily.

Building Long-Term Client Relationships

Follow-Up and Feedback

Post-Service Follow-Up: Send a follow-up message or call after the service to check on the client's satisfaction. This gesture shows you care about their experience and are committed to their satisfaction.

Encourage Feedback: Encourage clients to provide feedback on their experience. Constructive feedback helps you improve your services and shows clients that their opinions matter.

Loyalty Programs: Implement loyalty programs or offer discounts for repeat clients. These incentives encourage clients to return and build a long-term relationship with your barbershop.

Personal Touch: Remember details about your clients, such as their preferred styles, hair concerns, or even personal interests. Mentioning these details in future visits makes clients feel valued and appreciated.

Handling Difficult Conversations

Dealing with Dissatisfaction

Stay Calm and Professional: If a client is unhappy with their haircut, stay calm and professional. Listen to their concerns without interrupting and show empathy towards their situation.

Find a Solution: Work with the client to find a solution. This might involve adjusting the haircut or offering a complimentary service. The goal is to ensure the client leaves satisfied, even if it means going the extra mile.

Learn and Improve: Use feedback from dissatisfied clients as an opportunity to learn and improve. Reflect on what went wrong and how you can prevent similar issues in the future.

By mastering effective communication skills, barbers can build strong, trusting relationships with their clients. Thorough consultations, active listening, and professional advice ensure client satisfaction and foster loyalty, ultimately contributing to the barbershop's success.

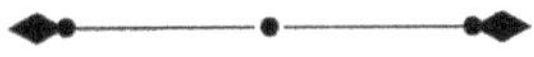

CHAPTER 11

MASTERING ACTIVELIS TENING FOR CLIENT SATISFACTION

Active listening is crucial in barbering, enabling you to understand clients' needs, desires, and concerns for outstanding results. By genuinely engaging with clients, you build trust, foster satisfaction, and strengthen relationships. Key techniques include maintaining eye contact, asking open-ended questions, reflecting and clarifying, observing non-verbal cues, and avoiding interruptions. These methods ensure you capture all relevant details during consultations, maintain ongoing dialogue during haircuts, and handle complaints effectively. Additionally, post-service follow-ups show clients you value their satisfaction beyond the appointment. Mastering active listening not only enhances client interactions but also contributes to long-term loyalty and success in your barbering career.

The Importance of Active Listening

1. **Understanding Client Needs:** Active listening allows you to truly understand what the client wants in their haircut, beyond the superficial descriptions. Clients may not always articulate their desires clearly, either due to a lack of technical knowledge or difficulty expressing their vision. By actively listening, you can interpret their words, tone, and body language to grasp the essence of their expectations.

2. **Building Trust and Rapport:** Clients appreciate barbers who genuinely listen to their input. When clients feel heard and understood, they are more likely to trust your expertise and judgment. This trust fosters a stronger barber-client relationship, encouraging repeat business and positive word-of-mouth referrals. Active listening shows that you value their opinion, making them feel respected and appreciated.

3. **Identifying Underlying Concerns:** Sometimes, clients may hesitate to express all their concerns

verbally. They might fear sounding critical or not know how to articulate their worries. Active listening helps you pick up on subtle cues and underlying concerns that may not be explicitly stated. This enables you to address potential issues proactively, ensuring a more satisfying experience for the client.

Techniques to Enhance Active Listening

1. **Maintain Eye Contact:** Maintaining eye contact shows the client that you are focused and engaged in the conversation. It conveys confidence and helps establish a connection. However, be mindful of cultural differences regarding eye contact, and adjust your approach as necessary.

2. **Use Open-Ended Questions:** Encourage clients to share more by asking open-ended questions. Instead of asking, "Do you want a trim?" try, "What kind of look are you aiming for today?" Open-ended questions invite clients to elaborate on their preferences and provide more detailed information.

3. **Reflect and Clarify:** Paraphrase what the client has said to confirm your understanding. For example,

"So, you're looking for a style that's easy to maintain but still has a bit of edge?" This not only shows that you are listening but also allows the client to correct any misunderstandings before you start the haircut.

4. **Observe Non-Verbal Cues:** Clients often communicate through body language and facial expressions. Pay attention to these non-verbal cues as they can provide valuable insights into their feelings and preferences. A client's hesitation or enthusiasm can guide your approach and ensure you meet their expectations.

5. **Avoid Interrupting:** Allow clients to express their thoughts without interruption. Cutting them off can make them feel rushed or undervalued. Practice patience and give them the space to communicate fully before responding.

Practical Applications in Barbering

1. **Consultation Phase:** Begin each appointment with a thorough consultation. Ask about the client's lifestyle, hair care routine, and any specific challenges they face.

This information helps you recommend styles that not only suit their preferences but also fit their daily life. During the consultation, apply active listening techniques to ensure you capture all relevant details.

2. **During the Haircut:** Continue the conversation as you work. Check in periodically to ensure the client is happy with the progress. For instance, ask, "How does this length look so far?" or "Is this the texture you were envisioning?" This ongoing dialogue keeps the client engaged and reassures them that their input is valued.

3. **Handling Complaints:** Active listening is crucial when dealing with complaints or dissatisfaction. Listen without becoming defensive, acknowledge the client's feelings, and clarify their concerns. Responding empathetically and making adjustments as needed can turn a negative experience into a positive one, demonstrating your commitment to client satisfaction.

4. **Post-Service Follow-Up:** After the haircut, take a moment to review the final result with the client. Ask for their feedback and express your willingness to

make any tweaks if necessary. Follow-up messages or calls can also show that you care about their satisfaction beyond the appointment.

Mastering active listening is essential for any barber aiming to provide exceptional service. By understanding client needs, building trust, and identifying underlying concerns, you can deliver haircuts that not only meet but exceed expectations. Implementing these techniques in your daily practice will enhance your client relationships, foster loyalty, and ultimately contribute to the success of your barbering career. Remember, a satisfied client is not just a one-time customer but a lifelong advocate for your skills and services.

CHAPTER 12

SKILL PRACTICING AND DEVELOPMENT

Developing your skills is essential for growth in barbering. This chapter will guide you on:

Practice Techniques Effective practice is key to mastering barbering skills. Here are various methods to enhance your proficiency:

1. **Using Mannequins**: Mannequins provide a risk-free environment to practice new techniques and styles. They allow you to experiment and perfect your skills without the pressure of working on a real person.

2. **Attending Workshops**: Workshops offer hands-on training with experienced instructors. They provide the opportunity to learn new techniques, stay updated with industry trends, and receive immediate feedback on your work.

3. **Practicing on Volunteers**: Practicing on willing volunteers helps you gain real-world experience. It allows you to understand different hair types and client preferences, improving your adaptability and confidence.

Essential Tools and Equipment Mastering the use of essential tools and equipment is foundational to a successful barbering practice. Here's what you need:

1. **Barber Stations and Chairs**:
   - **Barber Stations**: Invest in a well-designed station with ample mirrors, lighting, and compartments for easy access during haircuts.
   - **Barber Chairs**: Comfortable, adjustable chairs with hydraulic lifts, reclining functions, and headrests ensure client comfort and proper haircutting posture.

2. **Clippers and Guards**:
   - **Clippers**: High-quality clippers are vital for efficient and precise cutting. Choose between

corded and cordless options based on your preference and budget.

- **Clipper Guards**: A complete set of guards allows for various hair lengths and fading techniques. Ensure they are durable and fit securely onto the clippers.

3. **Shears and Thinning Shears**:

- **Barber Shears**: Invest in good shears for clean lines and precise detail work. Choose ones with a comfortable grip and appropriate size for your hand.
- **Thinning Shears**: These are used to remove bulk, create texture, and add movement to haircuts.

4. **Combs and Brushes**:

- **Cutting Combs**: Various combs are used for sectioning hair, guiding clipper and scissor work, and creating smooth transitions.
- **Styling Combs and Brushes**: These are used for finishing touches, blow-drying, and specific styles.

5. **Additional Barbering Tools**:

   o **Neck Strip**: For clean lines around the neckline and behind the ears.

   o **Straight Razor**: Optional but useful for close shaves and sharp lines (requires proper training).

   o **Clipper Oil and Disinfectant**: Maintain your tools by regularly oiling clippers and disinfecting equipment to ensure hygiene and optimal performance.

Choosing the Right Tools

1. **Quality Over Quantity**: Invest in high-quality tools that are durable and comfortable to use.

2. **Personal Preference**: Experiment with different brands to find the best fit in terms of weight, balance, and grip.

3. **Specialty Tools**: As you progress, consider adding specialty tools like texturizing shears to expand your skills.

Tool Maintenance

1. **Cleaning and Maintenance**: Follow manufacturer

instructions for maintenance, including oiling clippers and disinfecting equipment.

2. **Sharpening**: Have your shears and clippers sharpened periodically by a professional to ensure they deliver clean cuts.

Finding Mentors Learning from experienced barbers can accelerate your skill development.

1. **Finding a Barber Mentor**:

    o **Barber Schools and Instructors**: Seek guidance from instructors whose teaching style resonates with you.

    o **Established Barber Shops**: Look for reputable shops with experienced barbers known for their skills and mentorship.

    o **Industry Events and Competitions**: Attend events to connect with experienced barbers.

2. **Qualities of a Good Barber Mentor**:

    o **Experience and Skills**: A strong track record of success and recognized skills.

- o **Passion for Teaching**: Genuine passion for sharing knowledge.
- o **Communication and Feedback**: Clear, constructive feedback and a positive learning environment.

3. **Building a Mentorship Relationship**:

- o **Mutual Respect**: Value your mentor's time and expertise.
- o **Clear Expectations**: Discuss what you hope to learn from the mentorship.
- o **Open Communication**: Maintain open dialogue, ask questions, and actively participate.

Video Tutorials and Online Resources Online resources can further enhance your

skills.

1. **Advanced Haircutting Techniques**:

- o **Fading Techniques**: Master taper fades, skin fades, and burst fades.

- o **Texturizing Techniques**: Learn to add volume, movement, and style.
- o **Beard Shaping and Design**: Develop skills in beard shaping.
- o **Ethnic Hair Cutting**: Techniques for cutting ethnic hair textures.

2. **Online Resources for Barbers**:

- o **Online Tutorials and Courses**: Platforms offering tutorials and courses.
- o **Industry Websites and Blogs**: Stay updated on trends and techniques.
- o **Online Barber Communities**: Connect with other barbers and share knowledge.

3. **Utilizing Online Resources Effectively**:

- o **Evaluate the Source**: Ensure the credibility of online information.
- o **Combine Online Learning with Practical Experience**: Use tutorials to supplement hands-on practice.
- o Focus on Quality Over Quantity: Select the most beneficial resources.

Self-Evaluation Regular self-assessment is vital for continuous improvement.

1. **Tips for Self-Evaluation**:

   ○ **Regular Practice**: Dedicate time to practicing techniques.

   ○ **Seek Feedback**: Get honest feedback from clients and mentors.

   ○ **Record Your Work**: Film haircuts to identify areas for improvement.

   ○ **Set Goals and Track Progress**: Establish clear, achievable goals and track your development.

By continuously learning, self-evaluating, and refining your skills, you can establish yourself as a confident and proficient barber, capable of delivering exceptional haircuts and building a loyal clientele. This concludes Chapter 12 on Mastering Barbering Techniques. The next chapter will delve into essential business management skills for barbers, equipping you with the knowledge to build a thriving barbershop.